Step By Step

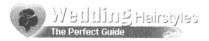

By Bella Darby
http://mybridehairs.com

Step By Step Wedding Hairstyles Copyright © MyBrideHairs.com

Table of Contents

Your Free Download

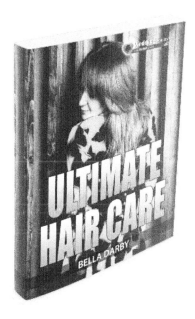

Get your free eBook called "Ultimate Hair Care" absolutely FREE!
Grab it now at http://mybridehairs.com/FREE

Disclaimer

No part of this publication may be reproduced or transmitted in any form or by any means, electronic or mechanical, including photocopying, recording, or any other information storage and retrieval system, without the written permission of the MyBrideHairs.com

This book is proposed for informational purpose only. The information contained in Step By Step Wedding Hairstyles, and its several complementary guides, is meant to serve as a comprehensive collection of time-tested and proven strategies that the authors of this eBook have applied to substantially increase their monthly passive income revenue on MyBrideHairs.com. All the images in the Books are taken from Wikipedia as source of education or from MyBrideHairs.com. Summaries, strategies, tips and tricks are only recommendations by the authors, and reading this eBook does not guarantee that one's results will exactly mirror our own results. The authors of Step By Step Wedding Hairstyles have made all reasonable efforts to provide current and accurate information for the readers of this eBook. The authors will not be held liable for any unintentional errors or omissions that may be found.

The material in Step By Step Wedding Hairstyles may include information, products, or services by third parties. Third Party materials comprise of the products and opinions expressed by their owners. As such, the authors of this guide do not assume responsibility or liability for any Third Party Material or opinions.

The publication of such Third Party materials does not constitute the authors' guarantee of any information, instruction, opinion, products or service contained within the Third Party Material. Use of recommended Third Party Material does not guarantee that your results, with (Title of website removed) will mirror our own. Publication of such Third Party Material is simply a recommendation and expression of the authors' own opinion of that material.

Whether because of the general evolution of the Internet, or the unforeseen changes in company policy and editorial submission guidelines, what is stated as fact at the time of this writing, may become outdated or simply inapplicable at a later date. This may apply to the MyBrideHairs.com website platform, as well as, the various similar companies that we have referenced in this eBook, and our several complementary guides. Great effort has been exerted to safeguard the accuracy of this writing. Opinions regarding similar website platforms have been formulated as a result of both personal experience, as well as the well documented experiences of others.

Introduction

Planning your wedding can be a very long and stressful process. However, whilst you are worrying about everything from the venue to the food, the groom's suit to the cars, you can forget any worrying where your wedding hairstyle is concerned. Every bride wants to be perfectly groomed on their big day and the hair style is a very important part of the grooming process.

Finding the right style for you can be quite a big task as there are so many to choose from and many of them depend on the style and length of your hair too. There are far too many to mention all at once, which is exactly why we have compiled a list of the latest and greatest hairstyles perfect for brides all over the world.

Required Tools & Products

Flat Irons
Hair Dryers
Curling Irons
Hair Brushes
Hair Combs and Picks
Hot Rollers and Hair Setters
Root Straightening Combs
Hair Clippers
Hair Trimmers
Shears
Hair Barrettes, Bands and Ties
Hair Extensions and Wigs
Salon Styling Hair Clips
Pouches, Mats, and Holders
Hair Dryer Attachments
Hair Towels and Turbans
Batteries, Chargers and Converters

Wedding Hairstyles for Long Hairs

(Method 1)

If you have long hair, it can often seem like a lot of work when trying to style it, so it's not hard to see why so many women with long hair worry about what to do with it for their wedding day. However, if you are one of these women lucky enough to have long hair, you are in a much better position than you think as long hair is most definitely easier to style than any other length. The fact that you have so much hair simply means that you can do so much more with it. If you are looking for something quick, easy and free for your wedding day hairstyle, this is the one for you!

1. Unlike most styles, you need to begin this one with hair that hasn't been washed for just over 24 hours. If you have naturally straight hair, you will need to add a few loose curls with your curling irons.

2. Then, add a little serum to make the hair a little easier to work with. Hair too silky and smooth is not easy to work with when doing this particular style. Once you have done this, separate the hair into three sections, leaving the slight majority at the back.

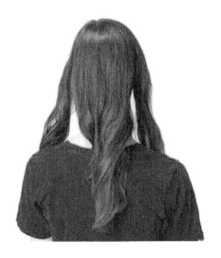

3. Take a small portion of hair from the larger back section right at the top and let it hang forward over your face. Then, take another section of hair from the back, roughly the same amount as the first section, and use your comb to back comb this section.

4. Then flip this section over on top of the first one. This will form the base of your new style.

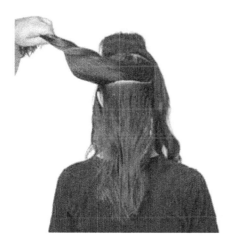

5. Now, take the final back section of hair and back comb it in the same way that you did the last piece. Now, flip the other two sections back over so they are in their original position at the back of the hair – all is it a little messier now!

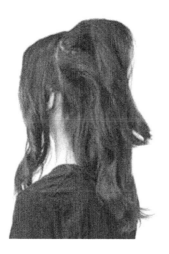

6. Taking care to smooth over any messy, frizzy parts of the hair, but not brushing out the back comb effect, take the hair from the back of your head and put it into a tight ponytail at the base of your neck.

7. Once you have done this, use the tail end of a tail comb to tease the ponytail and add volume to the style. The more you do this, the bigger your new do will be once completed.

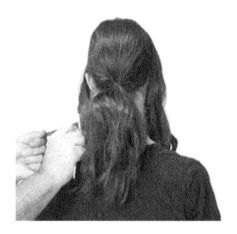

8. Take the ends of your newly voluminous ponytail and begin to twist it up and around, making sure you secure it with hair grips as you go.

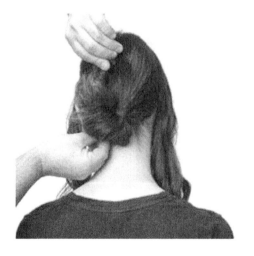

9. Once the bun/chignon has been put into place and secured with a few grips/pins, you can play with it a little with your tail comb to make it a little larger and looser. Once you have done this, give the hair a quick blast of hair spray for that little bit of extra security.

10. Now, starting with the left side of your hair split the side section into three individual sections. Take the one nearest to your bun and twist it around towards the back and secure it into the bun with a pin or two.

11. Repeat this step with the other two sections of hair on this side, wrapping them around the bun as you go.

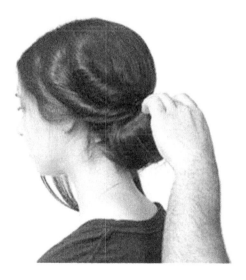

12. Now, take the hair on the other side of your head and split it into two sections, a top section and a bottom section. Back comb this hair in the same way that you did the back section and allow it to fall back into place at the side.

13. Now you can repeat the process that you did with the left side of the hair by twisting it round and wrapping it around the bun. Make sure all six of your side twists are securely in place with pins or grips and spray the hair with a little hairspray. Your look is now almost complete!

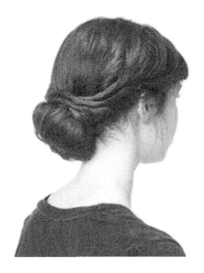

14. All that is left now is to add a few bits of sparkle to your new look. Add in grips with gems or pearls attached. This is a sneaky way to gain more security with your new style, all the while making the clips look just like an accessory.

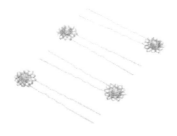

(Method 2)

Long hair can be difficult to style at times, especially if the hair is thicker than average. However, longer hair offers many more possibilities when it comes to a special new style for your big day. Follow the simple instructions below and create a whole new you for your wedding day. This look is a very simple one to achieve, however it will create such a classic bridal hair style in such a short space of time, it can save you two things so many brides are short of - time and money!

1. You can wash and blow dry your hair for this style if you prefer, but it does work best on hair that has not been washed for a day or so. If you choose to wash your hair first, when you blow dry, add in a little serum to give the hair some texture, making it easier to work with.

2. To begin with, use your curling irons to create a tight ringlet curl in your hair from around a quarter of the way down. This should leave you with the bottom three quarters of your hair in ringlets.

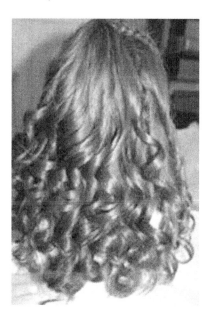

3. Now, comb the hair back from one side and fix it into a pony tail at the other side. This should create the look of a ringlet filled side ponytail with a sleek top. You will need to apply hair spray to the curls to ensure they don't drop and become loose through the day.

4. You can leave the style here if you choose to go for a more edgy look, but if you want something a little softer, continue reading. Using the tail end of a tail comb, pull the ringlets down and spritz occasionally with some shimmer mist or spray serum. This will loosen the curls and apply more of a wave to the style instead.

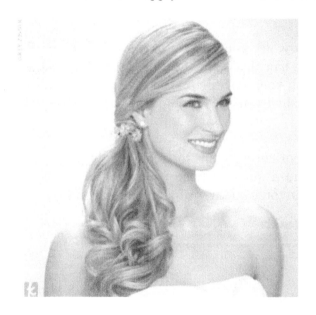

5. You can add looseness to the ponytail if you choose to add an even more relaxed look to this style. Finishing the style off with a large accessory like a flower clip adds something extra to this look and is perfect for weddings on the beach with a tropical theme etc.

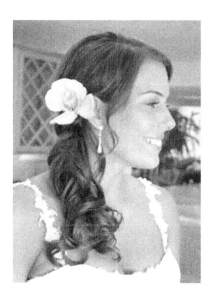

6. As a side note, if you choose to keep the ringlets and miss out the loosening step, you could avoid wearing the ponytail at the bottom of the neck and have it up high if you really want to make a statement! Again, add in some sort of clip, ribbon or flower to give it an extra something special.

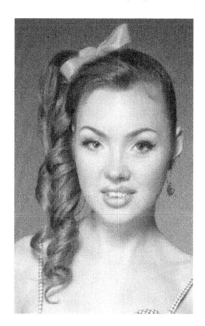

(Method 3)

A loose bun can be a quick way to get your hair up and out of the way ready to take the kids to school and get yourself to work, or even for wandering around the supermarket at the weekends. However, when done correctly, a loose bun can create a beautiful bridal style just perfect for your big day. Making a couple of simple little tweaks here and there can ensure you turn heads on your wedding day for all the right reasons.

1. Once you have washed your hair, dry it without using a blow drying brush. You don't want to create any kind of style or parting in the hair here. Now, add a little serum to your untamed locks and run a brush through it.

2. Now take the hair and fix it into a ponytail around 2 inches above the nape of the neck. If you create the ponytail too low down, depending on the size of your finished bun, it may touch your neck and will not sit properly when complete.

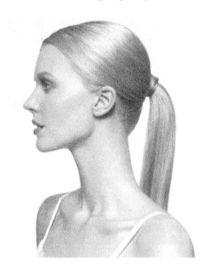

3. Now, take the ponytail section of your hair and twist it around from the tied end to the tips of the hair. Once you have the twist in place, wrap it around the bobble you have in, working out like a spiral design. Clip this into place with grips and pins as you go – you

don't want to use a bobble as this will show up when your look is complete.

4. However, you can use a bobble to secure the bun if you decide to use some sort of hair piece to cover it up when the style is finished. You should now have a fairly tight bun that doesn't really look like much at the moment!

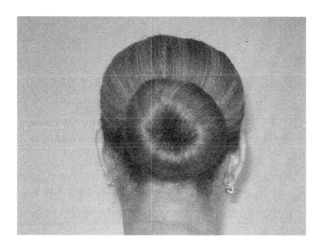

7. Once your bun is in place, you have the basis of your style completed. The rest is mostly down to personal choice now, so if you decide you like the look the way it is at any point, feel free to leave it like that. Take the tail end of your tail comb and poke it into the bun, loosening it up.

8. Make sure you spray with plenty of hair spray as you go – you want to loosen the bun without risking it coming apart completely! The bun is finished when you are happy with the style of it. We are aiming for an elegant, relaxed look here.

9. Take your time with this as you can loosen it up too much by trying to work too quickly. You can have the bun still fairly tight or with straggly ends hanging out – it is entirely your choice.

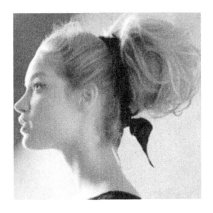

10. Once you have your bun the way you want it, and you have sprayed with plenty of hair spray to keep it secure, you are ready to make the finishing touches to your new style. Take a few strands of hair from the front at the sides of your hair and pull them down.

11. You don't really want to take down more than two or three from each side. Curl each one of these strands and spray them with hair spray. Now, just as you did before with the tail comb, loosen these ringlet curls into a loose wave.

12. This simply adds a more relaxed and beautiful look to this style and creates a certain flow to the hair. You can finish off your new bridal do with gems and crystals attached to hair grips or even a faux hair piece to go over your bun.

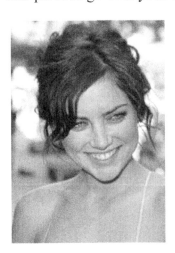

(Method 4)

If you are looking for something that appears spectacular and as though it has taken hours of a professionals time to achieve, this is very much the look for you. If you have long hair, you have the advantage of having more to work with and most of these intricate styles do require quite a bit of hair in order to get the desired effect. This style calls for freshly washed hair, so is best achieved after a wash and blow dry. Also, avoid using any products on the hair before you begin styling it.

1. Brush the hair back thoroughly to eliminate any knots or tangles. If you want a slightly outlandish look, you are going to need to focus your style to the top back section of your head, right where the crown is. If on the other hand, you require something a little more subtle and elegant, focus your styling a little lower down.

2. Brush the hair into a ponytail in your desired spot but instead of pulling all of the hair through as normal, tie the ponytail into a loop, leaving a long portion of the hair hanging down on the underside.

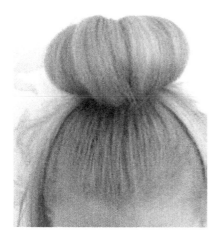

3. Now, wrap the dangling section of hair around the ponytail and grip it into place so that it resembles a loose bun. This piece will become the centerpiece of the bow you are creating. Using hair spray to set the style, separate the bun into two even sections, side by side

4. Use a mirror when doing this to ensure that your sections remain even. You can also use some hair gel when doing this part to set the hair even more. Simply rub a little bit into your hands before rubbing it onto the loose bun.

5. Try not to use too much as this can create a wetness of the hair which can be very difficult to work with. Set this part of the style with another blast of the hair spray.

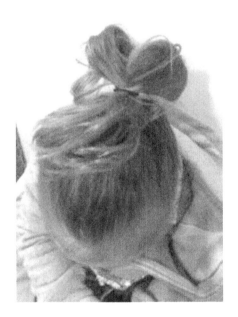

6. Now you need to take the loose strand of hair from the front and pull it back over the top of the two newly separated sides of your bun. Secure this in place with grips or pins and plenty of hair spray. You now have the basic shape of your bow.

7. Using a tail comb or even just your fingers, gently tease the sides of your new bow until they are fluffed out appropriately. This style shows a lot of personality so make it as big or as little as you like. Spray again with the hairspray one final time to set the look in place.

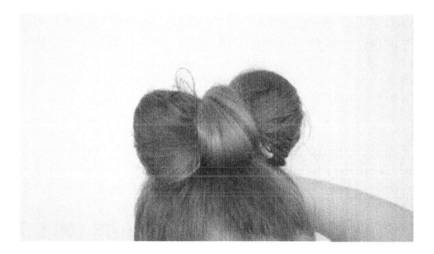

8. Finally, you need to secure the bow into the rest of your hair. Simply push a few hair grips through the sides of the bow and into the part of your hair that is up in the original bobble. Make sure you can't see the grips once they're in! You can also add sparkly gems and clips if you choose or just opt for some shimmer spray so that your hair catches the light and gives off a sparkle.

(Method 5)

You really don't have to spend hours (not to mention a small fortune!) in a salon in order to get a chic, beautiful and stylish look for your big day. So many brides book themselves straight into a salon without even considering the possibility of styling their own hair for their wedding day. Medium length to long hair means that you can do a lot more with your hair style than others and with just a few short minutes, you can create something that will dazzle your guests.

1. First of all, your hair needs to be freshly washed for this particular style, so wash and blow dry into a fairly straight style. You don't need to worry about any hair parting at all with this style.

2. Brush the hair through to get rid of any knots and tangles and fasten it into a standard ponytail a couple of inches from the nape of your neck.

3. Make sure your ponytail is in nice and tight to give you the right look for this style. If you want any straggling pieces of hair in your completed look, you will need to pull these down before you go any further.

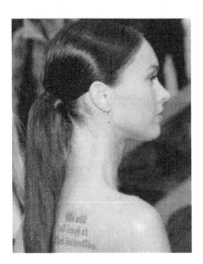

4. Now that your hair is up in a ponytail, you need to split the ponytail into two equal sections. Once you have done this, twist each side in the direction away from the ponytail right from the tip to where it meets the bobble. You can fasten the ends of your twists with clear bands.

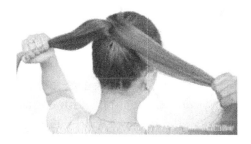

5. Now, twist your two twists together! Again, from the very end all the way to the top. Once you have done this, wrap the newly created twist around the bobble nice and tight, in the same way that you would for a normal bun.

6. Secure this in place with grips and then slick a little hair mousse on the top of your hair and spray your new twisted bun with plenty of hair spray. This look can be achieved in just a few minutes and costs hardly anything to create!

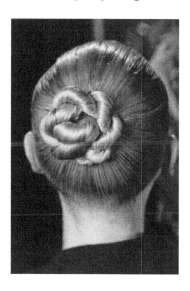

Wedding Hairstyles for Short Hair

(Method 6)

If you have short hair that you just can't seem to grow out into any kind of style. Fear not because you will not be stuck for style ideas on your big day. Hair extensions are a great way to add that extra length and volume to your hair for however long you wants it. However, long hair can take a lot of getting used to when you only really know how to style your own short hair, but don't worry; you're not going to have to pay a huge price for something you're going to see as a chore for weeks on end after your wedding day. You can get clip in hair extensions that will easily last the day and can be taken in and out as you choose. You can also style the hair extensions to suit the look you want to create for the big event! Putting in clip in hair extensions is a lot easier than most people think, so you don't have to spend a fortune on a hair stylist to do this for you.

1. Selecting your hair extensions.

You need to select the hair extensions that will best match the color and style of your own hair. First, choose the color – the assistant at the store will help you decide which the best match for you is. Hair extensions need to blend in with your own hair and therefore, give the effect of real hair, rather than looking like a weave or hair piece. Take note when shopping around – don't pay for cheap, imitation products – ensure your extensions are real human hair.

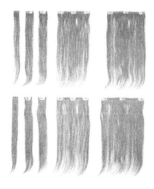

2. Styling your hair extensions.

If you plan to have your hair poker straight for your wedding day, you will need to straighten your hair extensions to match this. This works exactly the same way if you plan to curl your own hair. The hair extensions are real human hair, so you can style them in the same way you would your own, taking care to use heat defense spray to protect your new locks! To curl them, simply select a portion of the new hair, hold the curling iron in one hand and the hair in the other. Wrap the hair around the curling iron in exactly the same way you would do with your own hair and hold it there for around 10 seconds. Give it a quick blast of hair spray to set and release the hair from the curler. This should leave you with a tight ringlet curl. You can loosen this slightly by running the tail end of a tail comb through the curl once or twice. You can then add more hair spray to suit, and another spray would be better considering this is your wedding day and you really don't want your curls to start dropping out! You should be left with something resembling the photograph below. Repeat this for each section.

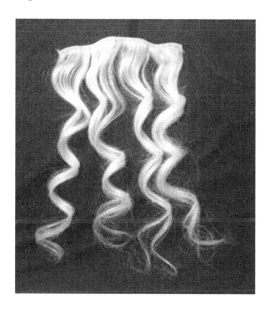

3. Preparing your hair for the extensions.

Once you have curled or straightened your own hair to match your new extensions, you need to separate a portion of your hair from the rest. Most packets of hair extensions you can buy come in sets of ten as pictured above. You can use as much or as little as you require to get the volume and length you are looking for. To begin, take a large portion of your hair from the top section, leaving just a small layer of hair around the back and the sides. You will need to do this for every large piece you have. For instance, if you plan on using three large pieces, you will need to do this three times. Therefore, select what you feel to be the right amount of hair each time for an even split.

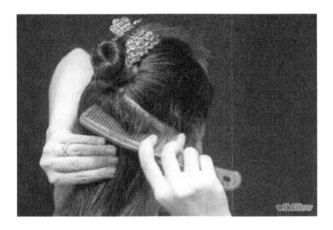

4. Inserting the hair extensions.

Once you have separated your first section of hair, you can begin attaching the first extension. As you can see in the photograph below, you need to hook the small clips onto your own hair. Gain a tight fit by clipping them to a few hairs on the top (put up) section of the hair as well as the hair that is down. This will ensure the hair stays put all day and doesn't simply slide down! Work by doing the back center first of all, and then move around the sides of the hair, making sure it is pulled taught, but just enough so there is not too much pressure on the extensions that they are pulling down on the hair.

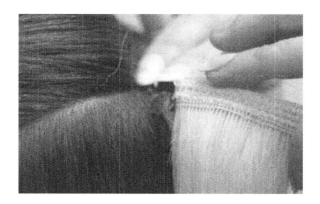

5. Inserting your side pieces.

Follow step four until you have inserted all of the large pieces that you intend to use for your new style. The more you use, the more volume will be added to your hair, but you will always achieve the same length. Once you have done this, you should be left with the sides of your hair looking a little limp compared the rest. This is where you are going to use the thin strips with just one clip, as shown in the first picture. Separate the sides of your hair into sections in the same way that you did for the larger pieces. Start with one side first and complete this before moving onto the next side of your hair. Insert the clips in exactly the same way, but using a much smaller section of hair each time, to suit the smaller section of hair you are trying to insert.

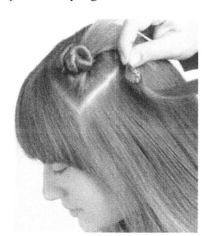

Once completed, play around with the hair until it sits right. You can run the tail end of a tail comb through it again to blend the extensions in with your own hair a little more until you complete the look you are aiming for.

(Method 7)

Many people with shorter hair often struggle to find a style suitable for their wedding day. However, whilst shorter hair does limit your choice compared with long hair that in no way means that you should be at a complete loss as to the style to choose for your big occasion. A classic look is what many women want on the day; something simple and elegant with a hint of sparkle. This can be achieved just as easily with short hair as it can with long hair. If your hair is shoulder length, or even in a bob of some kind, there is plenty of hair to work with for a nice bridal style that will wow your guests. Adding a few curls to sleek, straight hair gives a simple, classy look that you can embellish upon with gems and pearls.

1. Straightening your hair to a polished finish

Brush hair through thoroughly before straightening it and creating a slight inward facing flick at the ends. Make sure you use heat defense spray in order to protect your hair from the ceramic plates on your straightening irons. Separate the hair into sections with a clip, straightening each small section at a time in order to get full coverage with the straighteners and not leave any cheeky curls behind! Once it is all straight, apply a little serum to give the hair a shiny look and feel.

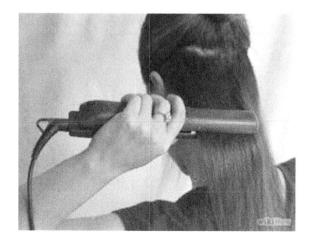

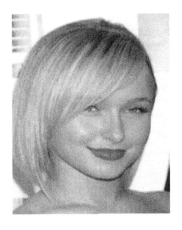

2. Mix it up a bit!

Once your hair is completely straight and you have used the serum to give it a shine, take a very small section of hair from the very top, about three inches away from the side of your face. Starting at the very top of the section, create a tiny plait with the hair and fasten the end with a clear band. Repeat this process with another section around two inches further back, and then do the same with the other side of your hair. Once finished, you should be left with four (or you can add more to suit your taste!) dainty little plaits, adding something a little bit different to your sleek look. The plaits should be small, like the ones shown in the picture below

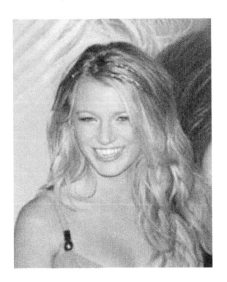

3. Add in some sparkle.

Once you have added in your little plaits, you have almost finished your new wedding day style. All that is left is to finish off your look with something sparkly to catch the eye. You can do this with small gem/pearl spirals. You can get these in the color of your choice and in a style that will suit your wedding day well. For instance, if your dress contains pearls, you may want to add the pearl style to your hair. These spiral clips are very easy to attach to the hair and your look can be completed in just a couple of minutes. If you want a very specific order to the gems or pearls, decide on exactly where you want them and place them symmetrically on both sides. However, a more wayward style is often better with these kinds of accessories. Placing four or five of them in a few different places around the hair adds just the hint of sparkle most bride's desire. Simply wind them round, working with the direction of the spiral design, until you reach the gemstone or pearl at the top, and the clip should be attached securely into the hair. You can also add a quick blast of hair spray to set the look for the day. You should now be left with a lovely end result, without having to spend hours or hundreds of dollars on your new style!

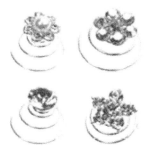

(Method 8)

Short hair styled into a bob may seem like a plain and simple do, however there are many ways in which you can style a bob and play around with it until you have a special new bridal style for your wedding day. If you are looking for something easy to achieve that will add a little sparkle and shine to what is most of the time a rather "normal" hairstyle, this is definitely the one for you.

1. First of all, separate the hair into two sections, putting the majority into a clip or bobble at the top of the head. Straighten the piece that is left down at the back and sides of the head. Repeat this process as many times as is necessary, each time leaving more hair down, until you have covered all of the hair. Remember to use some kind of heat defense spray in order to protect the hair from the ceramic plates on your straightening irons.

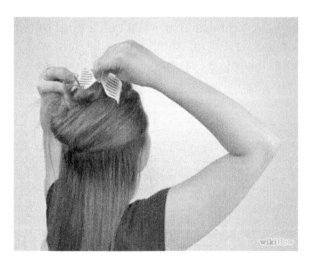

2. Apply serum to the hair in order to give it a shine. Only apply a very small amount if you're trying to achieve just a shimmer. If you want a complete wet look, apply more to suit.

3. Select a small portion of hair around three inches from the side of your face toward the back of your head. Use your straightening irons or a curler to add in a ringlet curl. Remember not to hold the curler

there for too long – you don't want to burn your hair! A quick blast of hairspray before releasing the curler will help to keep the curls from dropping throughout the day. Use the tail end of a tail comb to pull the curl down slightly and loosen it. Repeat this process as many times as you want to gain the amount of curls you would like. Anything from just two at the sides to 6 all over the hair will suit this style.

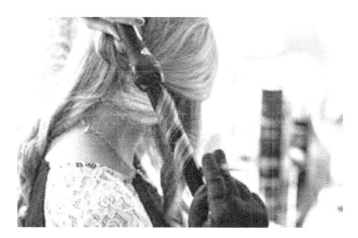

4. Once you have added in your required amount of curls, all that is left is to finish off your new look. A quiff adds something a little different to your style but is still a very simple look to achieve. Take a small section of hair from both sides and a little from the top. Comb the section of hair upwards so you are holding the ends of the hair above your head. Now, pull the hair back until you are pinching the very ends and holding them flat to your head where your hair parting is. Now you need to fix this into the rest of your hair with grips/pins or even a fancy clip.

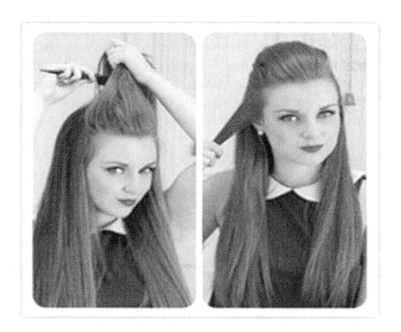

You should now be left with a sleek and sexy style that really doesn't take that much time to achieve!

(Method 9)

A bob can be the perfect style for you if you don't have much time for your hair on a daily basis. However, a bob can also be the perfect starting point for a beautiful new style for your special day. Implementing just a couple of tweaks can change your do completely from your normal every day look to a spectacular, new, fashionable bridal style.

1. Separate the hair into sections and straighten each portion of your bob, leaving a top section at the back, until you have covered it all. Take care to use heat defense spray to protect the hair too. Once the hair is poker straight, you could add some sort of shimmer mist to the hair to give it a sparkle when it hits the light. Just a couple of sprays at the front and back are required. You may not notice it straight away but when the mist catches the light it will give off a lovely effect. Once the hair is thoroughly straight, you are ready to move onto the next portion of the style.

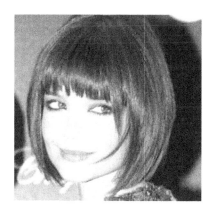

2. Take the straightening irons, and only on the top layer of the hair (no sectioning off needed now) curl the hair under, still leaving the piece at the back alone. Start at the side and working around the back of the head to the other side, take one piece at a time and clamp it into the straighteners, pulling the hair underneath towards the face (be extra careful with this part!). Make sure you only take a section no bigger than will fit comfortably in the straighteners; otherwise you will create kinks in the hair that will be difficult to undo. Once

completed, this will give the hair a flick underneath, creating an edge of classic style.

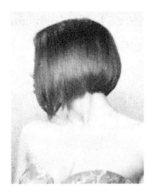

3. Now we are going to style the piece of hair at the back that has been previously untouched. You will need to get your comb and hairspray at the ready! Take a portion of the hair and, using your straightening irons, straighten the hair upwards so it is clamped into the straighteners up above the head. Now, working quickly, take your comb and pull the hair down out of the clamp of the straighteners. Do this until all of the hair is down again. Repeat this step until all of that section of the hair is done. Give this part of the hair a long blast of hair spray to thoroughly cover it. This should leave you with a large quiff and rather messy back section of the hair! Now, take the comb and hair straighteners and straighten this part of the hair, starting from the crown, no further up, until it is poker straight. This should leave you with a large quiff at the back going down into a poker straight style like the rest of the hair. This edgy and classic look is sure to turn heads on your big day!

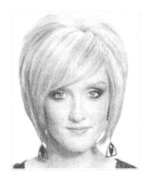

(Method 10)

If you have short hair and are looking for a special style for your wedding day, start looking back instead of forward! One of the most obvious times of beauty was the 1920's and the flapper girl style. This style may seem plain to some, but when your hair is a straight, simple shoulder length style it can be the something new you need! This look doesn't take very long to achieve and you certainly don't need to go and spend a week's wages in the salon either.

1. First of all, blow dries your hair into a side parting. If your hair usually parts in the middle, this may feel a little strange for a while, but you will soon get used to it. Comb the hair down so that it stays put. If you get a few strands of hair that don't want to stay in their new position, apply a very small amount of serum to encourage it! As your hair is relatively short, you will have a large portion at the front that is shorter than the rest of the hair on its new side. Use a clip to keep this in place for now.

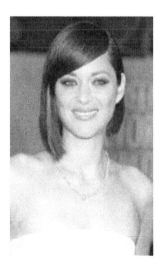

2. Section off the hair ready to straighten it. Make sure you leave the parting at the side. As you go around the hair to straighten it, don't clamp the hair from the root to the very ends as you normally would. Only straighten from the root to around half way down. If your hair is shoulder length, straighten to roughly the top of the ear. Take the

section of hair you clipped to one side and straighten that piece from root to tip. Then, clip it back where it was for now. You can now apply as much serum as you require giving the hair a sleek finish.

3. You should now be left with half straightened hair, and the bottom half in its post blow dried, pre styled state. Now, take your curling irons (or you can use your straighteners to curl the hair if you prefer) and curl the bottom half of the hair, all of the way around. Once this is completed, you should be left with hair that is straight on top, and a mass of ringlets at the bottom. Make sure you spray your new curls with hairspray to avoid them dropping out throughout the day. You can also either curl the ends of the side swept "fringe" that you kept clipped away earlier or leave it poker straight. Either way, you will need to clip the ends underneath that side of the hair, using the rest of the hair to hide the clip.

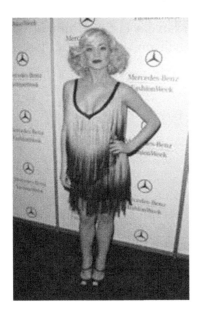

5. Play with your curls until you achieve the look you desire. You can leave the curls tight and full or you can use the tail end of a tail comb to pull the curls down and loosen them slightly. Now, it is time to glam up your new do even further with spiral gems or similar. Spiral gems are always a good choice as they are cheap to buy, easy to put in and add that little bit of sparkle that most brides are trying

to achieve. Simply work with the spiral design of the clip and attach the gems into the hair. A great place to put these would be right at the top of the curls, just where they start as you will have a ledge of sorts to work with. This should leave you with a timeless, classy style that is sure to turn heads!

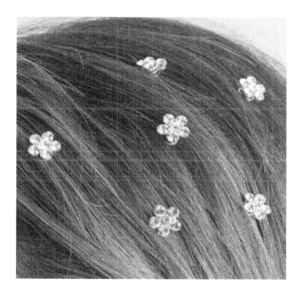

Half up Half down Wedding Hairstyles

(Method 11)

Half up half down hairstyles give a classic look in a quick and simple way. There isn't a large amount of time required to achieve this look, nor do you need to pay top dollar for a qualified stylist to do it for you. No doubt your wedding day has already drained your bank balance so cutting costs wherever possible is probably on your never ending to do list!Try out this super quick style for a timeless look on your special day.

1. Make sure your hair is freshly washed and blow dried ready for this style. Don't dry the hair until it is bone dry however, as a little damp to the hair will help you to achieve the look we're aiming for here.

2. Add some mousse to the hair and run it through with your fingers. Take some large rollers and roll each section of the hair up towards the nape of your neck. Clip each roller section into place with a grip or hair pin and be careful not to roll them too tight. Only do small sections of hair each time, otherwise your it will not fall into the desired style well. Add a couple of blasts of shine spray once the rollers are all in and allow them to set. It can be useful to use some sort of loose shower cap at this point to keep any hairs from going stray out of their rollers!

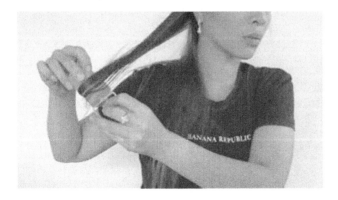

3. Blast the rollers all over with the hair dryer for a couple of minutes and then leave them to cool down and dry completely before removing. When you are taking the rollers out, be careful you don't pull the hair and get it caught in the roller. Take your time and persevere – it will all be worth it!

4. Once all of the hair has been removed from the rollers, run your fingers through it gently. Flip your hair forward, tipping your head upside down and give it a quick flick around to allow the waves to fall evenly. Be careful not to play with the hair too much as this is a sure fire way to lose your new look and make it go limp.

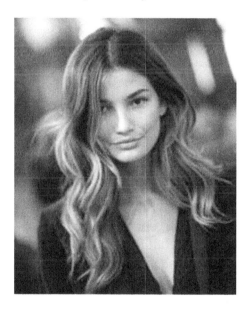

6. Now, take a small section of hair from each side of your head, making sure you've made an even selection. Clip one side up with a grip or pin and start with the other side first. Plait the hair in the same way you would with any other standard plait and pulls it round towards the back of your head. Clip it into place with some bobby pins. Now do the same with the other side. Give the hair some more shimmer spray and a touch of hair spray if you feel you need it and voilà! You have a sexy, free flowing style with waves polished to perfection.

(Method 12)

This style is one you can have much more say in. You can decide upon wavy, curly or straight hair to begin with and what size you want the main feature to be. So, to begin with straighten or curl all of your hair. It is best to do this style with freshly washed hair that has been thoroughly dried.

1. Now, select a small section of hair from each side of your head. The larger the section you choose, the larger the main feature will be.

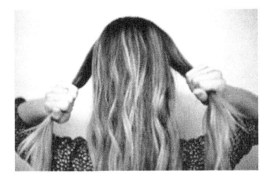

2. Tie both of these sections together with a bobble or band and put the hair into a ponytail. Don't pull the ponytail all the way through – leave it with some hair dangling out in the shape of a loop.

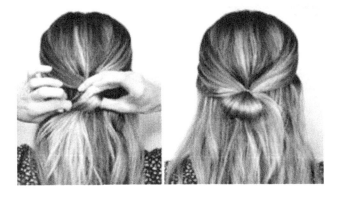

3. Pull the loop into two equal separate sections with your fingers, leaving you with two loops. Use a grip or hair pin and clip one loop to the side until later.

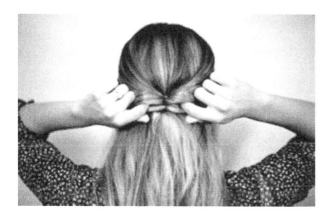

4. With your first loop, spread the hair out with your fingers to make a large bow shape and use a grip to set it in place. Grip from the bottom to the top (the inside of the bow shape) and then grip from the top to the bottom. This will ensure it stays secure.

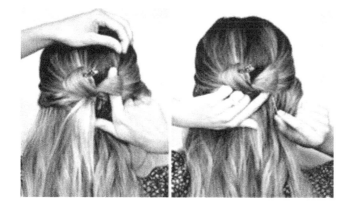

5. Simply repeat the previous step with the section you clipped away earlier to complete the bow shape.

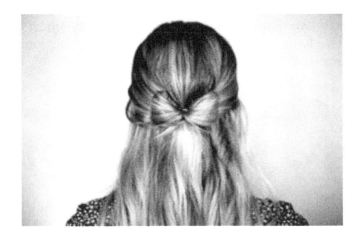

6. Now, for the final step, take the remaining ponytail hair that is still dangling down and wrap it around the bow elastic until it is no longer showing. Grip this hair into place underneath. Now, give the hair a quick blast of hair spray and then a little shimmer spray to finish off this sleek bow style.

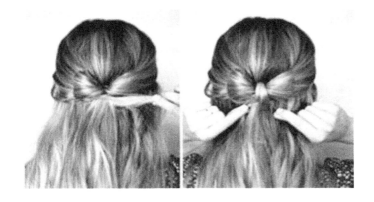

(Method 13)

Half up half down hair styles are a very popular choice for anyone on their big day. Whether your hair is long or short, thick or thin makes no difference at all – you are sure to be able to find a style to suit you. The following style is a very simple yet classy look that will turn heads on your wedding day for all the right reasons! You can add in accessories to suit as you go and there really is no limit to what you can do with this particular look. If you want to change things up a little as you follow the step, and then do so – this is your special day and your hair should look exactly as you want it to.

1. Take a curling iron or straightening iron and gently tease the ends of your hair to create a large wave or a loose curl. Make sure to use heat defense spray when you are doing so in order to protect your hair.

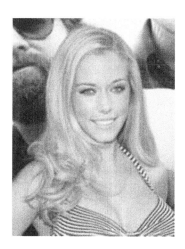

2. Once you have curled the hair, take three large sections off the top and clip them to keep them separate from the rest. Bring the left section round to the right hand side, creating a large quiff of sorts at the side of the head. Fix this in place with hair grips or pins. Now, do the same on the next side, bringing the hair from the right hand side of the hair over to the left hand side. Again, fix this in place with grips or hair pins. Once sides are done, take the large section from

the top of the hair at the front and bring this back, giving a large quiff at the fringe area.

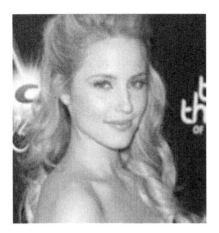

3. Once you have completed the above two steps, give the hair a few squirts of hair spray to set your new style in place. You could also add some spiral gems to the hair for a little added sparkle if you choose to.

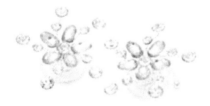

(Method 14)

The following half up half down hair style is ideal if you are looking for something simple to achieve, yet beautiful and classy looking for your big day. Ideal for medium to longer length hair, this hairstyle is quick and easy to do but leaves the hair in the perfect bridal style. Sure to turn heads, this hair style will leave you feeling like a princess on your wedding day

1. Leaving a large top section of hair pinned away, use your hair straighteners to get the hair into a loose curl all the way around. Always make sure you use heat defense spray to protect the hair when curling. Run the tail end of a tail comb through the hair when the curling is completed to ensure the curls are not too tight. This should leave you with more of a rugged wave. Scrunch some hair mousse into this to set the style once finished.

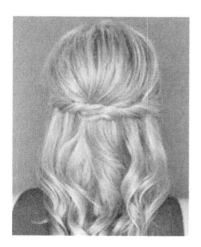

2. Take the large portion of hair that was pinned back and back comb it with your comb. When this is done, fold it back and use hair grips to pin it in place at the back of the head. This should leave the hair with a large quiff at the top.

4. Now, take two pieces of hair, one from each side and twirl them in towards the head. Cross them over when you get to the back of the head and pin them in place. Super easy!

5. If you wish to hold the style securely as most people do, you can add a few sprays of hair spray to the hair or scrunch some more hair mousse into the ends. To give the hair a nice sparkle when it catches the light, add some shimmer mist to the finished style.

(Method 15)

Half up half down hair styles are perfect for brides. One of these stylish looks can be achieved easily with little time and no need to go to the salon. The morning of your wedding can be so stressful with so much to fit in it seems impossible to get it all done in one day! Therefore, cutting out the usual requirement of a trip to your stylist can be a godsend. The following style is very easy to achieve but does not look that way when complete.

1. Style the hair into loose curls with your curling iron or straighteners. Tease the curls with the tail end of a tail comb to ensure they are not too tight when done. Add some texture spray to the hair and a little hair spray if you wish.

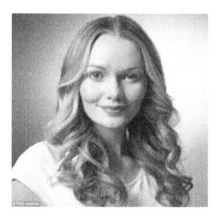

2. Gather up a large chunk of hair from the crown of your head. Take care to leave a good amount at each side, as these bits will eventually make your braid. Back comb the large piece of hair you have separated at the crown, pressing the hair down at the bottom into the scalp. Now, gather up this portion of hair into a quiff style shape and smooth out the top with a comb. Once smooth, pin the hair in place at the back of the head with two hair grips.

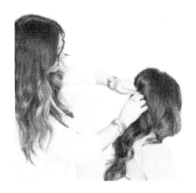

3. Take one of the sides you left with free hair and braid the hair down. Leave out any hair that you want to have framing your face when the style is finished. Once the plate is done, pin it to the back of the head with hair grips, covering the main quiff you started with. Now, do the same with the free hair on the opposite side of your head. Once done, pin this over the top of the first braid. Tuck the dangling hair down underneath the plait of the first braid.

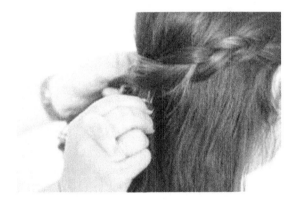

4. Spray the braids with enough hair spray to lock the style in place but don't add too much as this can make the hair hard and rough to the touch. You can easily add a pretty tiara or headband to this look to finish it off if you require.

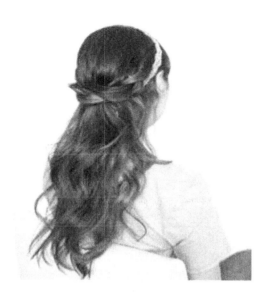

Curly Wedding Hairstyles

(Method 16)

Curly hair has a very romantic look to it. When looking for a wedding day hair style, it is important to select one that fits well with the look you are trying to achieve. Whether that is something plain and simple or something extravagant and glamorous, there is a hair style out there for you. The following style will add to any classy, beautiful bridal look and will make a feature of your curls so much that nobody will be able to take their eyes off you!

1. Begin this style with freshly washed and dried hair. Try to leave the hair to dry naturally to give your curls their full bounce, but if this is not possible for you, make sure to use heat defense spray. Coat your curls with a texture gum or hair mousse to smooth them out and eliminate any frizz that may appear after washing.

2. Take a section of hair from the top of your head, as if you were preparing for a half up, half down style. Clip or tie this hair in place over to the right hand side of your head. Release a small section at a time – you will make up around 12 sections all together when finished. Twirl this section around, going backwards towards the back of the head. Grip the hair in place just behind the ear. Repeat this step with all sections of the hair going all the way around until you reach the other side of the head.

3. Cover the grips you have put in with spiral hair clips or hair pins with gems attached. This should completely cover the grips so nobody can see them, even up close. It will also add a pretty diamante or colored gem to the base of each twist and create a very modern, sparkly look!

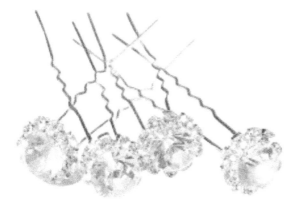

4. You will need to spray the hair with plenty of hair spray now to keep the style from slipping out at all throughout the day. It is also a good idea to take a few spare spiral clips with you in your bag just in case!

(Method 17)

Bridal hair styles do not have to be sleek and sophisticated to look good. There have been and will always be a great number of more glamorous brides, and if that's the look you're hoping to achieve for your big day, the following style oozes glamour, making you look gorgeous and sexy in a modern, tame and beautiful way. Very quick and easy to do, this style will make you look as though you have just stepped out of the salon and spent hundreds on your new look. This look works well with both straight and curly hair but the hair needs to be of a relatively long length – don't worry though, extensions are fine to use!

1. Brush the hair through thoroughly to get rid of any tangles or knots. Once you have done this, brush it all back and apply a little hair mousse or texture gum with your hands.

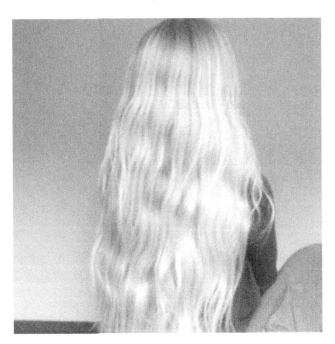

2. Back comb the top section of hair with a ratting comb until it is all done. Now, smooth it over with a soft bristled brush, making sure to

leave some of the rugged style in place. Once completed, sweep all of the hair over to one side.

3. Now that the hair is swept fully over to one side, separate a chunk of it. If all the hair is sitting over your right shoulder, take the chunk from the left. The section of hair you have separated will become the bobble around the rest, so choose the size according to what you want from the finished look.

4. Pull the large portion of your hair into a bobble style and wrap the smaller section around it in a side ponytail at the nape of the neck. One you have done this, pin the "bobble" section of the hair underneath with grips or hair pins so that they are made invisible. You will need to use two or three.

5. Simply spray the hair all over with hair spray and lift it with the tail end of a tail comb anywhere you want to create a little more bounce.

(Method 18)

The following hair style is ideal for any bride on her wedding day, but is particularly suited to those with long, curly hair. It is perfectly fine to use hair extensions and the hair will need to be in rather thick curls before starting. This look is a very chic and sexy one, glamorous but in a very tame way. Sure to wow your guests, this new look will truly leave you feeling like a princess on your special day. Follow the steps below to achieve this quick and easy style. All you will need are curling tongues, a few hair grips or pins, a ratting comb, hair spray and any accessories you wish to add to the hair when the style is complete such as hair pins with gems or a large flower to sit at the side.

1. Take a small section at the top of the hair, going no further back than halfway between the crown and the hairline. Just as if you were about to create a half up half down look

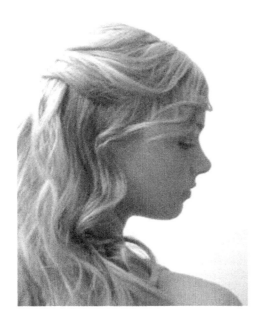

2. Now, separate this new top section of hair into three and clip the two side pieces away for later. Take the center piece of the top

section and back comb it with your ratting comb. You can add some hair mousse here to make this a little easier, but this is non-essential.

3. Now, allow the back combed hair to fall back into its original position and smooth it down with a soft bristled brush. You don't want the hair to be too high, but it needs a little bit of a lift. Now, take the two side pieces of hair that you clipped away earlier. Bring these around to the back and, going over your back combed area, cross them over each other. Grip the ends in place with a couple of hair grips or pins and add a quick blast of hair spray to lock it in place.

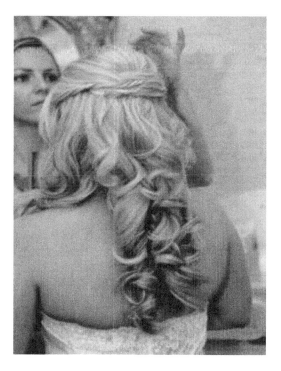

4. You can now add any accessories you like, from diamante hair pins to a tiara. Finish the style off in any way you choose to put your own stamp on it.

(Method 19)

The following style will definitely wow the guests at your wedding reception. If you want a new look that is traditionally bridal, looks as though you have spent hours in a salon, but is actually relatively quick and easy to do yourself at home, this is the look for you. Follow these simple steps and achieve a true fairy-tale wedding hair style with no fuss and no bill! This one is for those with curly hair; however you don't need to have natural curls to make it work.

1. Start this style with hair that has been freshly washed and dried thoroughly. Brush it through well and ensure you remove any knots and tangles. If your hair becomes frizzy once dried, add a little shine serum to it to smooth it out.

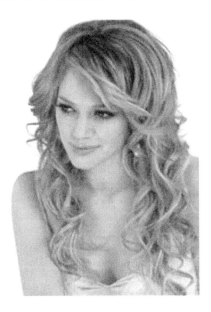

2. Now, place the hair into a high ponytail, leaving a few pieces dangling free that will later be used to frame the face. If you have a fringe, leave this free as you can style this is the usual way at the end.

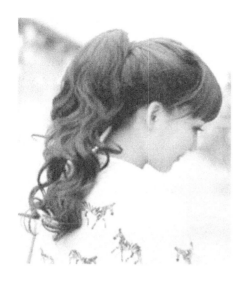

3. The hair that is dangling out of the ponytail is going to be your main focus now. Take small pieces at a time, and clip them all over the hair, around two inches away from the base of the bobble. As you move through the hair, allow the pieces to overlap each other to create a "messy" bun.

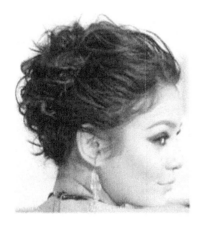

4. Now that the main part of the look is complete, take any small strands of hair that are hanging loose (aside from a couple to frame the face) and pin them back to the top of the head, near the top of the new bun. Add in any accessories you like to finish the style off. Pearl and diamante clips work well, and a tiara always sits nicely

with this style. This part is entirely up to you, and is your way of incorporating your own look into the style.

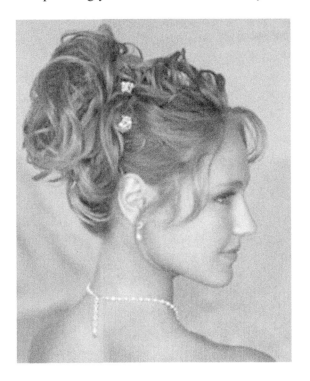

(Method 20)

Ombre hair extensions are incredibly popular at the moment with women all over the world, including some of our most loved celebrities. This look can of course be achieved with your own hair, however if you do not wish to damage the natural hair with coloring products or you simply only want this look for your wedding day, hair extensions are definitely the way to go. The hair extensions (clip-in style) are attached in exactly the same way as normal and can still be curled to match your own hair. The steps below will show you how to turn plain hair extensions into ombre hair extensions quickly and easily with a home dye kit and a tinting bowl and brush.

1. Hair extensions cannot be bleached and therefore, if you are looking to dye the ends of dark extensions blonde, you will need to rethink this. The best way is to choose a set of blonde hair extensions that will become the ombre part of the hair and dye the top section to match your own hair colour.

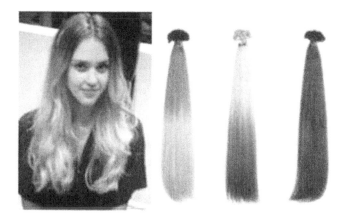

2. Brush the hair extensions through thoroughly to remove any knots or tangles that may be in them. Then, lay them down on an old sheet or just use a surface that you don't mind getting some hair dye on!

3. Brush the hair dye onto the extensions with the tinting brush. Make sure you coat them thoroughly and only go halfway down.

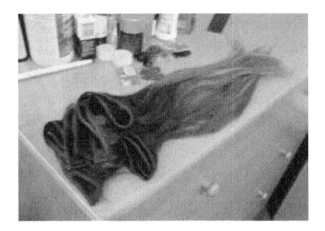

4. Leave the dye to set for the recommended amount of time. Once enough time has elapsed, you will need to prepare the hair for rinsing. Apply plenty of conditioner to the ends of the hair before rinsing as this will help to stop the color from running through the non-dyed section. Now, simply rinse the dye out and apply some shampoo and conditioner in the same way you would do with your natural hair.

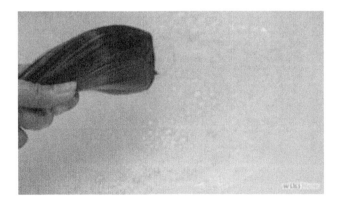

6. Leave the hair to dry naturally (you should always do this with extensions) and then curl them to suit the natural style of your own hair before applying. This should leave you with a great set of ombre

hair extensions that will look great on your wedding day with any style you choose to put them in.

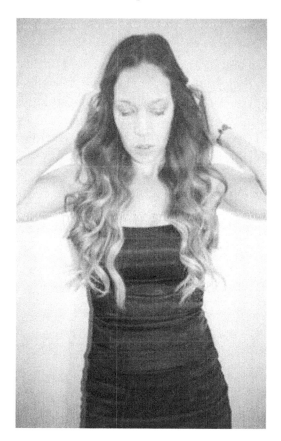

Wedding Updo hairstyles

(Method 21)

The French twist is a very chic and classy look for a bride. For those women wanting a beautiful and elegant look for their big day, this is definitely a good choice. Quick and simple to achieve, this style will sweep the hair away from the face and frame it wonderfully. Best of all, this look can be done in the comfort of your own home without the need to spend money out of the wedding budget at a salon.

1. Brush the hair through thoroughly to get out any knots. Once this is done, comb or brush the hair entirely to one side, and pin the side swept part in place in a zigzag fashion with hair grips.

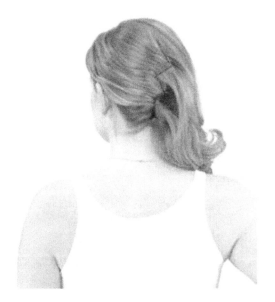

2. Now, once the hair is all pinned in place at the side, take the large section of hair dangling down and roll it all inwardly, twisting it towards the grips.

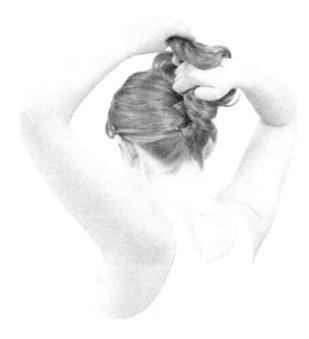

3. Grip the French twist in place by inserting grips through it at the side and into the hair underneath.

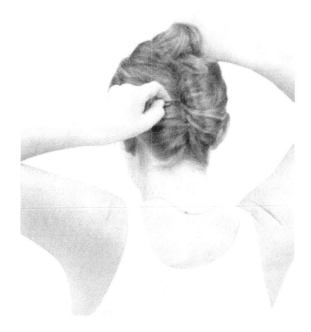

4. Spray the twist with plenty of hairspray to help set the style in place. Now, what you do with the hair that you are left with at the top is entirely your choice. You can choose to tuck it into the top of the twist and pin in place, but some people opt for a more wild and windswept look with the hair poking out at the top. Whichever you choose, make sure to add some hairspray when you're done. If you choose to, you can pull down a few strands of hair from the sides of the head, just above the ears, and curl them with your straighteners/curling irons to get some hair framing the face nicely.

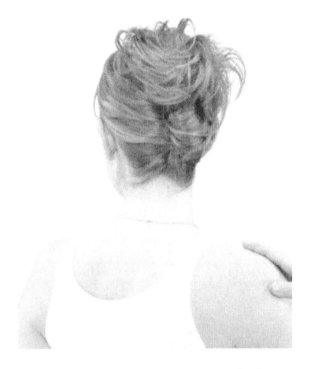

5. Adding accessories to your new look is one of the most important steps. You could go for gem encrusted spiral clips or pins with diamanté at the ends. If you are planning to wear one, a tiara or head dress would also suit this style well.

(Method 22)

The following style is a very classy look, with a very modern appeal. Giving a very elegant finish, this style suits many women, younger and older alike. Give it a try and see if you want to make it your own for your big day. Bridal hair styling can cost an absolute fortune and an awful lot of your precious time on your wedding day morning, so styling your own hair quickly and easily into a fantastic finish can be a great way to save time and money!

1. Begin with hair that has just been washed and dried. Allow the hair to dry naturally if you can, but otherwise make sure to use heat defense spray of some kind to protect the hair from the dryer heat. Brush the hair through thoroughly and back comb the top, back section a little to create some bounce. Smooth the back combed section down with a soft bristled brush, being careful not to push it down to the scalp.

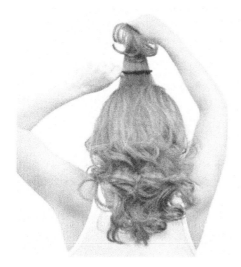

2. Separate the hair into three equal sections at the back and put it into a plait as normal. Leave a little hair loose at the end of the plait.

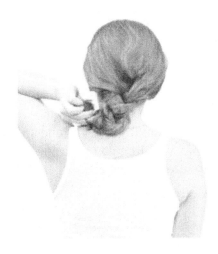

3. Curling the plait around to the left take the loose hair at the end of the plait and wrap it around the plait, tucking it into one of the gaps. Use a hair grip to pin it in place underneath the plait where it can't be seen. This should leave you with a rather rugged looking braided bun. You can now play with it as much or as little as you like. You could pin different sections in to make it very tight and neat or loosen small pieces of hair in the bun to create a more windswept style. You can also add any gems or clips you like to the bun or the hair at the top of the head.

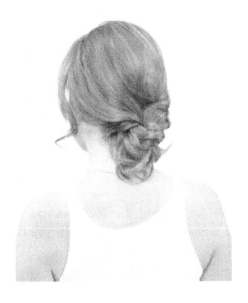

(Method 23)

Many women unfortunately believe that to get a classy, sleek style for their hair on their wedding day involves a long trip to the salon and spending a small fortune. However, this is simply not the case anymore. You can easily create the perfect bridal style with little time and effort required and certainly no big cost to consider. Follow the steps below and see if you can complete this style to the standard required for your big day. Remember – practice makes perfect!

1. Begin with hair that hasn't been washed for around 24 hours or so. Brush it through well, and separate it into two sections, the top one slightly smaller than the bottom one.

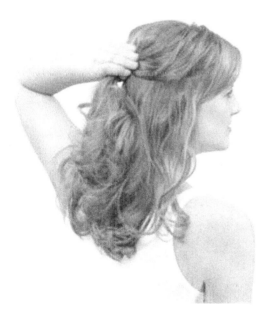

2. Now, separate the top section of hair into two equal pieces and tie them together to form a simple knot. Insert a couple of hair grips to hold the knot in place, leaving the ends to dangle down.

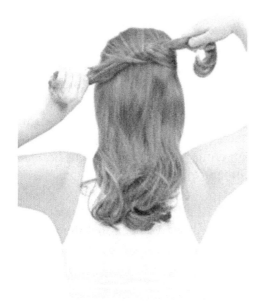

3. Now, with the free hair at the bottom of the head, separate into two sections again. Repeat the above step and knot the hair in the middle, again pinning it in place with grips. Do the same knot again with the hair left at the nape of the neck, each time leaving the ends of the knots to dangle down

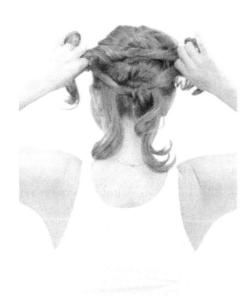

4. Choose any two of the knots on the right hand side of the head and tie them together in another knot. Pin this in place with two hair grips, one going from bottom to top and the other from top to bottom. Do the same with any two knots on the left hand side of the head.

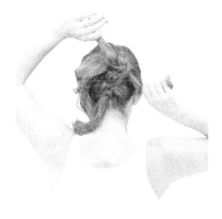

5. Pin up any loose ends of hair and grip underneath where the grips will not be seen. Spray a little hair spray on the hair in order to hold the new style in place, and you should be left with a stylish knotted bun! You can pull down any hair at the front to curl or wave in order to frame the face.

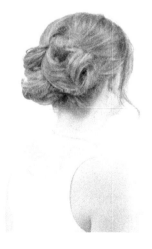

(Method 24)

When it comes to a beautiful bridal hair style for your wedding day, many women believe that they need to go all out and create a new and spectacular style in order to stand out and look fantastic. However, this is not true at all. You can take a relatively well known and well used style and create something a little different with it, adding little twists here and there to make it extra special for you. The following style is one that many people wear day to day, but with a little time and effort, can be made into something very beautiful indeed.

1. Place the hair into a ponytail, quite far down the head. You should add a little mousse or texture gum to the top of the hair here to smooth it down.

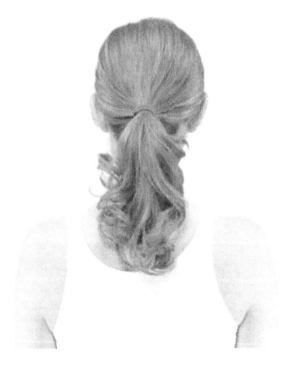

2. Insert your fingers into the hair just above the bobble. Try not to push the bobble too far down when doing this.

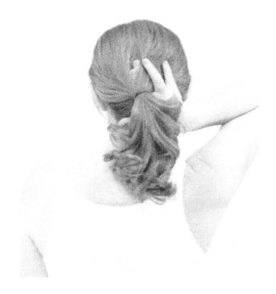

3. Lift the ponytail hair upwards and fold it under, tucking it down into the hole you have just made with your fingers.

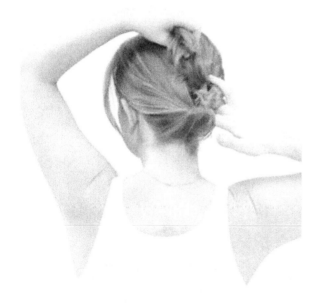

4. Now, pull the ponytail down and to the sides to tighten the style.

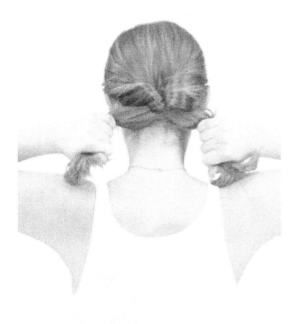

5. Smooth the hair at the top of the head into the twist with mousse. You can either leave the dangling hair in its natural style or you could add curls or waves to it. Add some hair spray to the style now to lock it in place. You can also bring down a few pieces of hair from the sides at the top and just above the ears in order to frame the face.

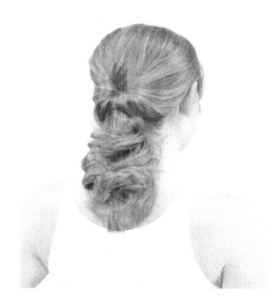

6. This style suits a tiara very well, but if you are not looking to go down that path on the day, you could use other methods or decoration. Use accessories like spiral clips with gems and pearls attached (to suit your look and theme) or maybe a large flower pinned into the side of the hair. This part is entirely up to you and your individual styling choices.

(Method 25)

Many brides to be believe that the hairstyle they choose for their big day must be utterly perfect, symmetrical and polished to perfection. This is simply not the case. Some of the most beautiful and sophisticated styles that can be achieved for a bride are rather wayward in appearance and give off a windswept look. This kind of hairstyle is now becoming more and more popular with women all over the world that want to create a more natural look for their wedding day. The following style is a very relaxed and rugged one, yet still looks incredibly beautiful as though it has taken hours when in reality it has only taken a few minutes!

1. Curl the hair completely; separating the hair into sections as you go to ensure it is all done properly. Once finished, run the tail end of a tail comb through each curl to loosen them into more of a natural wave than a styled curl. Now, spray with some hair spray to lock the waves in place. Make three chunky plaits in the hair, one at each side and one at the back.

2. Brush the hair back pulling the plaits to the back too, taking care not to brush out the waves too much. Don't worry if the hair looks messy at the top! Just make sure it is all flat to the head! Tie all of the hair, plaits included, into a ponytail just above the nape of the neck.

3. Twist the ponytail hair around loosely and pin it as you go into a loose bun shape around the bobble. Make sure it is all pinned in securely with hair grips or similar. Give it a long spray of hair spray to secure the style. You should now be left with a very relaxed, loose bun that oozes sleek and sexy!

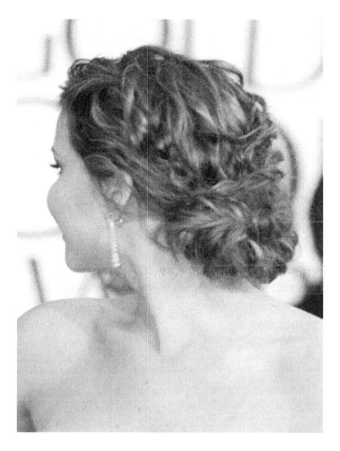

4. Some nice gems and diamantes would go well with this style, adding a little more sparkle to it. Due to the plaits at the front, a tiara is not completely out of the question, but it is also not really suited to this style.

Vintage Wedding Hairstyles

(Method 26)

The vintage look is a beautiful one indeed, especially when done for a bride. More and more people nowadays are looking to the past for style ideas for their big day, and for good reason too. So many of the timeless, classic styles created way back when are still used by brides today to create the elegant, perfect look they are hoping to achieve on their wedding day. If you are going vintage for your bridal style, try out this authentic look to wow your guests.

1. This look is best achieved with hair that has not been washed for around 24 hours. If you feel you must wash your hair, make sure it is thoroughly dry before beginning the style and add a little texture gum or hair mousse before starting.

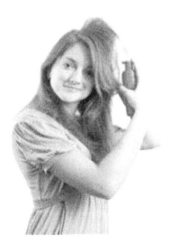

2. Back comb the hair all of the way around, leaving a small section at the front that will become a side swept fringe. Make this back combed hair into a quiff style at the front, pinning it in place with hair grips. Now, do the same around the sides, pinning/gripping as you go. Then, tie the hair into a bobble, pushing the quiff up and making it even larger.

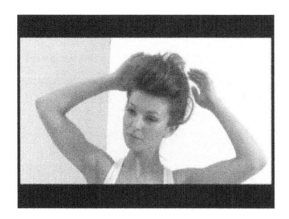

3. Before moving onto the next step, ensure you have sprayed the hair well with hairspray in order to help lock your new quiff style in place. Now, tuck the hair in the ponytail into the original bobble, creating a loose loop. Alternatively, if your hair is long enough, you could create a loose bun. Now, sweep the front portion of hair over to create a side fringe and pin it in place behind the ear with a hair grip. This hair style is often very well matched with a small head band or fascinator to set the look.

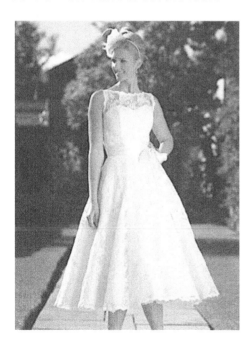

(Method 27)

The vintage look is one that many more women are now adopting, specifically for their wedding day. Most people feel that a bridal hair style should be elegant and sophisticated, beautiful and glamorous. A vintage wedding day hair style can be the perfect solution for any bride struggling with the decision of how to have her hair on the big day. So many "new looks" are in fact not new looks any more, but old looks that have been reinvented by people time and time again to create modern day twists on vintage styles. The following style is one that is easy to create, yet boasts a certain Hollywood feel and is sure to wow your guests.

1. Begin this style with freshly washed hair and ensure it is dried thoroughly before starting. Brush the hair through well with a good brush.

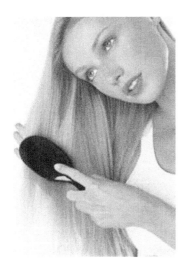

2. Create a side parting in the hair at whichever side feels best for you. Using 1 inch curling tongues or hair straighteners, curl small sections of the hair one at a time. Once a section has been curled, clip it to the top of the head with a hair grip or pin. Wait until each piece is completely cool before removing the grips and allowing the hair to fall naturally.

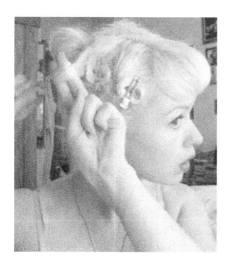

3. Add a little bit of hair spray to the hair but be careful to only use a small amount as using too much on this style will make the curls hard and crunchy. Add a little shimmer spray to suit your style and away you go!

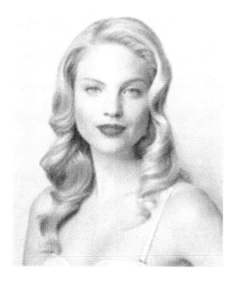

4. To finish the style off and add a little something special, you can use hair clips with gems and diamanté stones on them. It is also entirely possible to wear a tiara with this style or even some large, decorative flowers in the hair.

(Method 28)

Having a vintage look for your wedding day may seem quite daring but, when done correctly, is very much worth it! One of these gorgeous old styles can be perfect for any bride that really wants to turn heads on her big day. Whether you are looking for a very over the top costume style or something quite a bit more subtle, the vintage look is definitely one to try out.

1. Begin this style with freshly washed, thoroughly dried hair. Brush it through well to eliminate any knots and tangles. Now, part the hair in the center and leaving a small chunk at the front (each side), brush the rest back. Tie the brushed back portion of hair into a ponytail.

2. Now, take one of the side pieces (clip the other for now to keep it out of your way), and run the straighteners down it. When you get to the tip of the hair, twist the straighteners slightly to create a kink at the bottom of the hair. Now, spray this chunk with hair spray and comb it through. Then, back comb it and smooth it out with hair wax/texture gum.

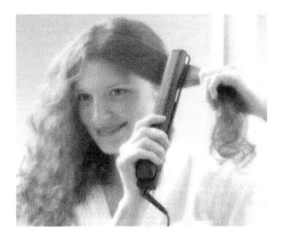

3. Once the section of hair has a kink at the end, wind it around your fingers (two fingers should be enough). Wind it up and pin it to the top of the head with two or three hair grips. Now smooth over the victory roll with some hair spray or texture gum rubbed into your

hands. Now, repeat this process with the other chunk of hair you clipped away earlier. You should now be left with the perfect victory rolls placed on top of the head.

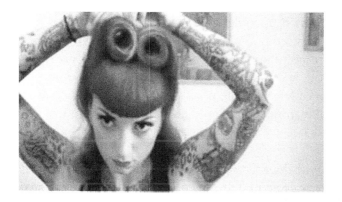

4. The final step is simply to style the rest of your hair so it falls how you want it to. Leaving it poker straight is of course an option, however many brides prefer to add some curls. You can choose to curl just the ends of the hair or ringlet the hair from root to tip – entirely up to you.

(Method 29)

The 1960's beehive has been a very popular style ever since its inception. Made famous by people such as the Ronnette's, this style remains well used to this day. A bridal style can be anything from subtle beauty to extreme glamour and a vintage look is a great way to get the best of both worlds. The beehive look can be done in a more relaxed style in order to create a subtle look and back combing into a huge quiff at the front will of course make it much more of an outgoing look.

1. It is best to start with hair that hasn't been washed for around 24 hours. To begin this style, curl the entire head of hair with a large curling iron. Make sure each section is complete and leave it to cool completely before moving on to the next step.

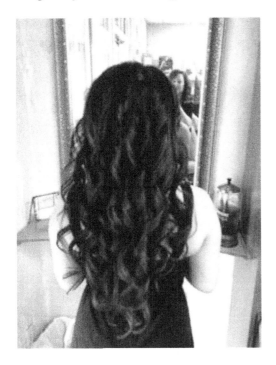

2. Making your way through the entire crown of the head, back comb all of the hair at the top with a ratting comb until it is as high

as you want the finished look to become. Leave out a small curl at the front to frame the face.

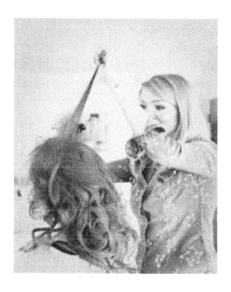

3. Now that your hair looks very ratty on the top, the style is beginning to take shape. Take some hair from the very front (still leaving out the accent curl) and smooth this hair down over the back combed part so it covers it well without pushing it down. Now, take some hair from each side and, smoothing it down as you go, pull this around the quiff to the back of the hair. Twist the hair around and clip together at the back with a few grips/hair pins. Arrange the ends of the twists nicely into vintage pinned curls. Now, pin a few small curls up behind your hair and into the main twist. This narrows the style somewhat and gives it a very authentic look. Finally, simply pin the accent curl to the chosen side of your head and spray with plenty of hair spray!

(Method 30)

A vintage hairstyle is a look that many women are now trying to achieve. Every bride wants to look special on her wedding day and no matter whether it is a big, fairy-tale wedding or a small gathering of family and friends, looking the part really do matter. The right hair style is an important factor in the brides look on her wedding day and can really make her style. The following look is vintage inspired and will most certainly wow your guests on the big day should you choose to use it. The following style is very sleek and elegant and will leave any bride looking beautiful on her big day.

1. Start this style with freshly washed and blow dried hair. Don't blow dry the hair straight, just let it fall naturally or even better still, leave it to dry naturally with the sun.

2. Sweep the hair back into a low ponytail and ensure the top of the hair is completely smooth with no lumps of bumps. You can add some mousse or hair spray if you like, but be careful not to use too much as this can make the hair appear greasy.

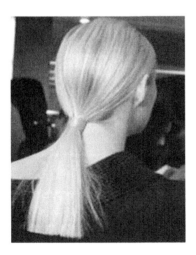

3. Now, take your curling irons or straighteners and make large curls within the ponytail. You may need to push the bobble up and tighten

it a little when you are done due to the curlers pulling the hair down but this is fine.

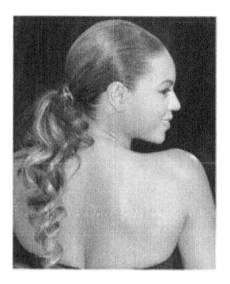

4. Now, starting from the very side of the ponytail with the curl the furthest to the left, begin pinning the curls up. If you have rather long hair, you can pin the curls halfway up and then fold them back down on top of themselves, pinning them once again at the bottom. Once finished, you should be left with a very vintage looking bridal style.

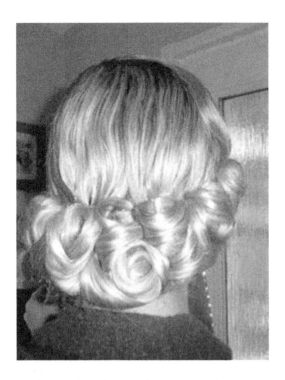

5. If your hair is not long enough to reach all of the way around your head, you could also split the hair into three low ponytails at the start (even sections, side, back, and side) and curl from there, following the same steps.

6. A tiara or head dress would be a nice touch with this look as it is very plain at the front, all of the focus being at the back of the head. You could also add in some diamante pins to the curls themselves once they are pinned up.

Indian Wedding Hairstyles

(Method 31)

Everything about an Indian wedding from the cake to the decorations is extravagant and beautiful. The bride's hair should of course follow suit. With many Indian women choosing to grow their hair out to a lovely long length for their wedding day, it is much easier to create a gorgeous new style for the big day. If you are looking for a bridal style that you can create yourself without having to pay the fee of a hair stylist, the following may be perfect for you.

1 Start this style with freshly washed and fully dried hair. Apply a little mousse to the hands and slide it through the hair. You can use texture spray if you prefer. You can also apply directly to the hair line and pull it down through the hair.

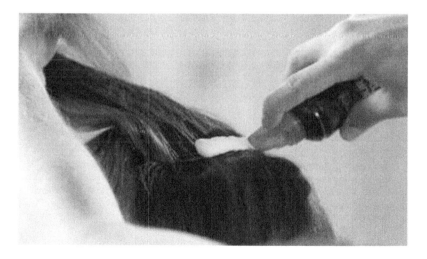

2. Take your curling irons or straighteners and create tight ringlet curls in your hair from just below half way down the head. Curl the hair in very small sections so that the ringlets are individually very small and tight. Give the hair a long blast of hair spray in order to lock the curls in place.

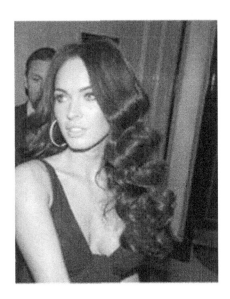

3. Sweep the hair back into a fairly low ponytail, a couple of inches from the nape of the neck. Be careful not to pull out any of your new curls during this part!

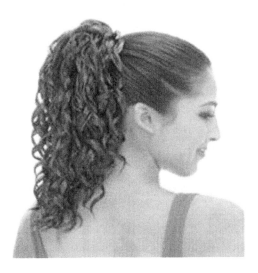

4. Now, you will need a small crocodile clip for the hair for this part. Take the ponytail curls and starting at the bobble, twist the hair a little until you have enough to put into the small clip. Now, clip the hair up to the top of the head and allow the small, tight ringlets to fall back. You can also use grips if you don't have the clip required.

This will give you the same finished result but may take quite a lot more time. Now, smooth over the top of your hair with mousse and give it a blast all over with some hairspray and shimmer spray to make it sparkle. This should leave you with a beautiful new bridal style in no time at all!

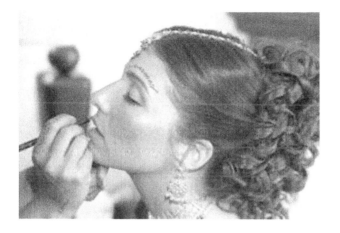

(Method 32)

Indian bridal hairstyles can be absolutely beautiful when done properly. Whenever they are seen, most people believe the bride must have spent hours in a salon and spent hundreds to get her hair to look so perfect. However, the fact of the matter is that you too could have that same perfect hair on your wedding day, with no need for hours in a salon and without a huge dent in the wedding budget. The following style is very classy and sleek and takes no time at all to achieve! You will need nothing more than a hair doughnut, a comb, two bobbles and some hairspray.

1. Starting with freshly washed and dried hair, add a little texture gum or hair mousse to make the hair easier to work with. Now, place the hair into a high ponytail, in exactly the same way you normally would.

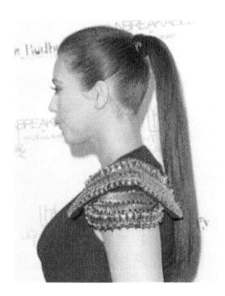

2. Take the hair doughnut and place it onto the ponytail, directly around the bobble.

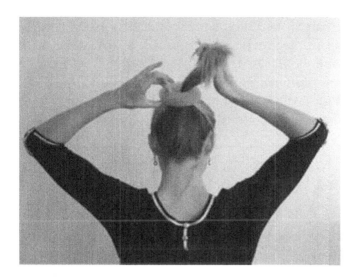

3. Now, take the hair in the ponytail, and insert your fingers through it so that you can feel the inside of the bobble. Spread the ponytail hair all around so it is evenly spread over the doughnut. Using both hands, pull the hair into the bun shape that is now beginning to take form and place your second bobble over it. You should now be left with the perfect bun shape, but with a lot of excess hair dangling down (depending of course on the length of your hair). Spray some hairspray on the style now to allow the bun to set. This way, you shouldn't end up with stray hairs falling out of the bun as the day goes on.

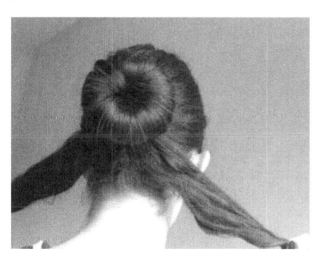

4. Now, wrap the hair around the bun so the ends finish underneath and pin everything in place with hair grips. This way, none of the bobble or doughnut should be seen. Give it one last blast of hair spray and add some shimmer spray to suit. Mousse over the top of the hair again to ensure a sleek finish and there you have it – a beautiful new bridal style in no time.

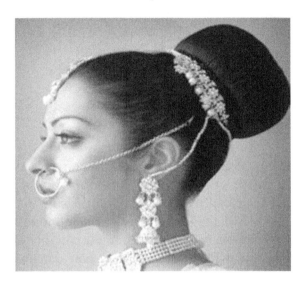

(Method 33)

Traditional Indian hairstyles are still extremely popular with today's brides. However, the younger generation is now looking to experiment with new looks and beautiful bridal styles to really wow their wedding guests. The following style is simple, yet classy and will be sure to turn heads on the big day. This style requires long hair, however extensions are perfectly fine to use. Giving a modern twist on an old hair style, this look is easy to achieve without the help of a hair salon.

1. This look is best started with freshly washed hair that has been fully dried. Part your hair in the center. Now, leaving a couple of inches at each side still parted, brush the rest of the hair back.

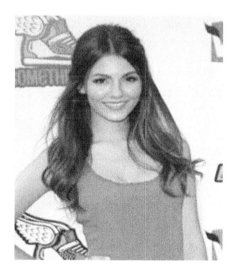

2. Now, braid the brushed back portion of the hair, making sure the plait is very neat and tight. When complete, tie the end of the braid with a clear band and spray with a little hairspray to avoid any loose hairs coming free.

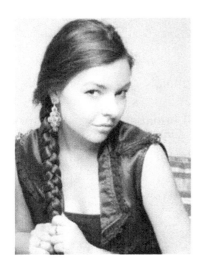

3. Just as you would put your hair into a bun normally, pull the braid around itself into a bun shape. Secure it as you go around with hair grips or pins. Try to make sure the pins cannot be seen. Give the hair another long blast of hairspray now. You can also add shimmer spray if you like.

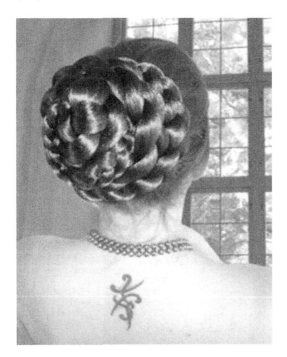

4. For the final step in this style, add a little sparkle! You can use hair pins with gems attached in order to lock the style in place further, adding in a touch of sparkle and shine as you go! You can also add the traditional Indian head wear too as it will fit nicely down the original parting you made in the hair.

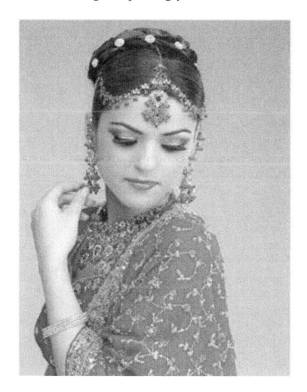

(Method 34)

Certain Indian hairstyles have remained popular for years and years and never seem to go out of fashion. The following style is one that many brides are adopting for their big day in order to achieve a classy and beautiful style with little time and effort. There is so much to do on the morning of your wedding that having a hair style that takes little time to put in place can be a great way to give yourself a little more time on the day.

1. This style is best achieved with hair that hasn't been washed for 24 hours or so. Begin by parting the hair in the center and leaving a couple of inches parted at each side but brushing the rest back.

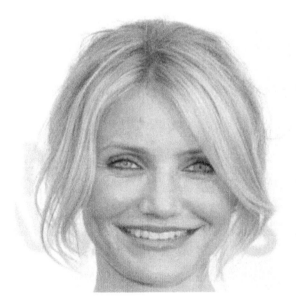

2. Now, back comb the large portion of hair that has been brushed back as if styling a quiff, adding a little hair spray as you go. However, don't pin the quiff in place with any hair grips; just leave it to hang down at the back.

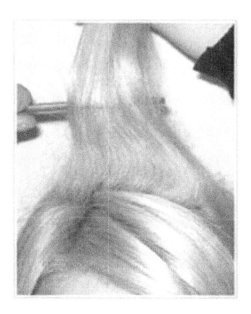

3. Once all of the hair has been back combed, place it into a tight ponytail, leaving the quiff to stand up at the front. Don't place the ponytail too high up the head and spray it with plenty of hair spray to lock the style in place.

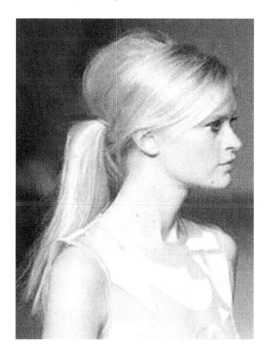

4. Now, take your curling irons or straighteners and curl the hair that is left hanging out of the ponytail. Spray with hair spray to hold the style and add shimmer spray to suit your own personal taste. You can now add any head dress or diamanté clips to suit your style. You could add a couple here and there, wear a traditional Indian head dress on its own, or go all out and cover your quiff in spiral gems.

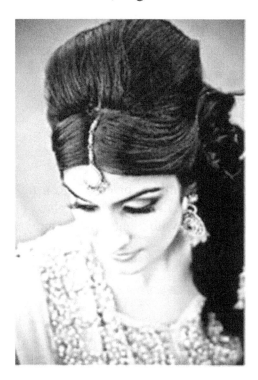

(Method 35)

Indian brides quite often wear a netted dupatta and due to the almost transparent material, the hair needs to be styled well as it will be seen through the netting. It is quite common for brides to want a fairly modern day style or even a traditional style with a modern day twist, yet include the Indian head wear such as a maang tikka as standard. Therefore, it is always best to create a hair style where the maang tikka can sit easily. The following style achieves a classic Indian look with a very modern twist.

1. Begin by braiding in a few very small plaits into the hair. Then, tie a bobble in the hair, around half way up the head, including the plaits. Leave out a couple of inches at each side of the head and make these into a center parting – this will make it easy for the maang tikka to sit nicely at the front.

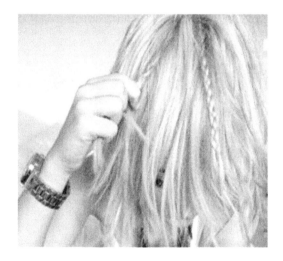

2. Now, using a hair doughnut (or not if you feel comfortable without one), create a bun in the hair. Apply a little hair spray or mousse to the top of the hair to smooth it out and spray on a little shimmer spray to suit.

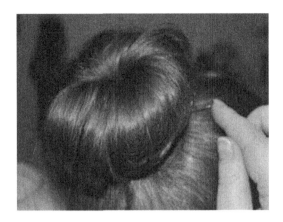

3. To finish off this classy new style, add the head dress, allowing it to sit in the center parting you created at the start. Now, you can either add lots of little sparkle clips/gem encrusted spiral clips or simply add one large one at the back center of the bun. This will make the new look even more special and perfect for a bride on her big day. Use hair grips to cover any loose bits of hair coming out of the bun, and pin them underneath so they can't be seen.

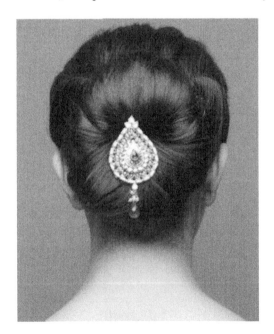

Your Free Download Again

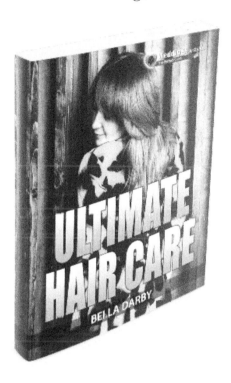

Get your free eBook called "Ultimate Hair Care" absolutely FREE!
Get it now at http://mybridehairs.com/FREE

About Bella Darby

Hi there, my name is Bella Darby. I am hairstylist with more than a decade of experience, a successful business women and mom of two lovely kids. I have experience of working in more than fifty saloons. I also help to create great hairstyles for weddings, parties and other functions occasionally. I got selected three times as best hairdresser in the yearly competitions.

I feel proud on how life taught me great things and prepare me to face the critical time. Few years later I completed my college I got married with my high school sweetie. Later, I went through a tough time in my life. I was homeless and bankrupt since my husband loss his job in financial crisis. Hence, I tried to get a job to support my family. After few weeks of job hunting I get a chance to work in saloon. I have learned great hairstyles while working in saloon.

I started part time hairstylist business once I got the good experience in my day job. Now that I am pretty much stable and support my family, I have started my own business of saloons. I have seen the struggle behind getting that best hairstyles and healthy hair. Hence, it has planted an idea in my mind to provide solutions via my site & books. I am pretty sure that my books are my best work reflection and knowledge which can help to achieve a needy a great hairstyle and healthy hair.

Note from Author

Reviews for this Book are gold to me! If you've enjoyed reading this book, would you consider rating and reviewing it? All I can offer you a FREE download for your honest review for this book. Please find your free download link given in this book.

To give your review, click here http://mybridehairs.com/Add-Review.

More Books by Bella Darby

Ultimate Hair Care
Reverse Hair Loss
Choosing Wedding Hairstyles

Get complete list at http://mybridehairs.com/books/

Thank You

Thank you for taking the time to check out my work. I hope you enjoy reading it as much as I enjoyed writing it! Authors wouldn't be anywhere without readers like you, so your support REALLY means a lot. I'm a firm believer that books don't need to be expensive or difficult to get hold of, so I want to encourage EVERYONE to enjoy the pleasure of books and not just mine.

Visit my website http://mybridehairs.com

Find me on other platforms:

http://www.facebook.com/WeddingHairstyles
http://twitter.com/WedHairStylez
https://plus.google.com/+Weddinghairstylez/posts
http://www.pinterest.com/wedhairstylez/

Made in the USA
Monee, IL
03 March 2023

29038476R00066